D. J.'s Happy Teeth

A Dental Health Book

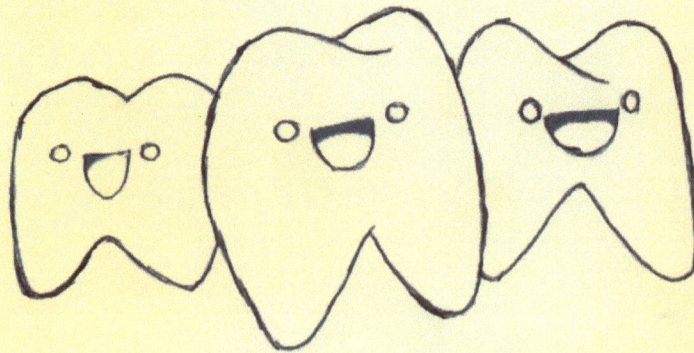

BY: KATRINA DEAS, RDH, MBA

ILLUSTRATED BY: EMILY KING

This is a story about a little boy named D. J. who has a very vivid imagination. He loves to smile and show his teeth because he has the most beautiful, perfect teeth for a six-year-old.

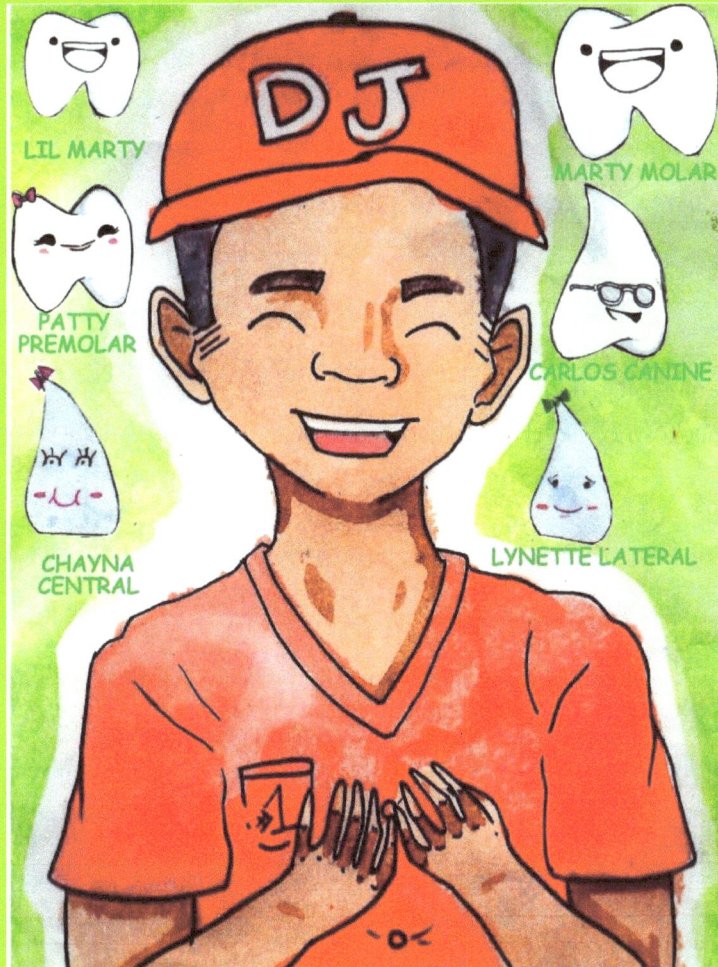

As D. J. got ready for bed, he started to get excited because he was getting ready to see twenty-four of his best buddies in the world.

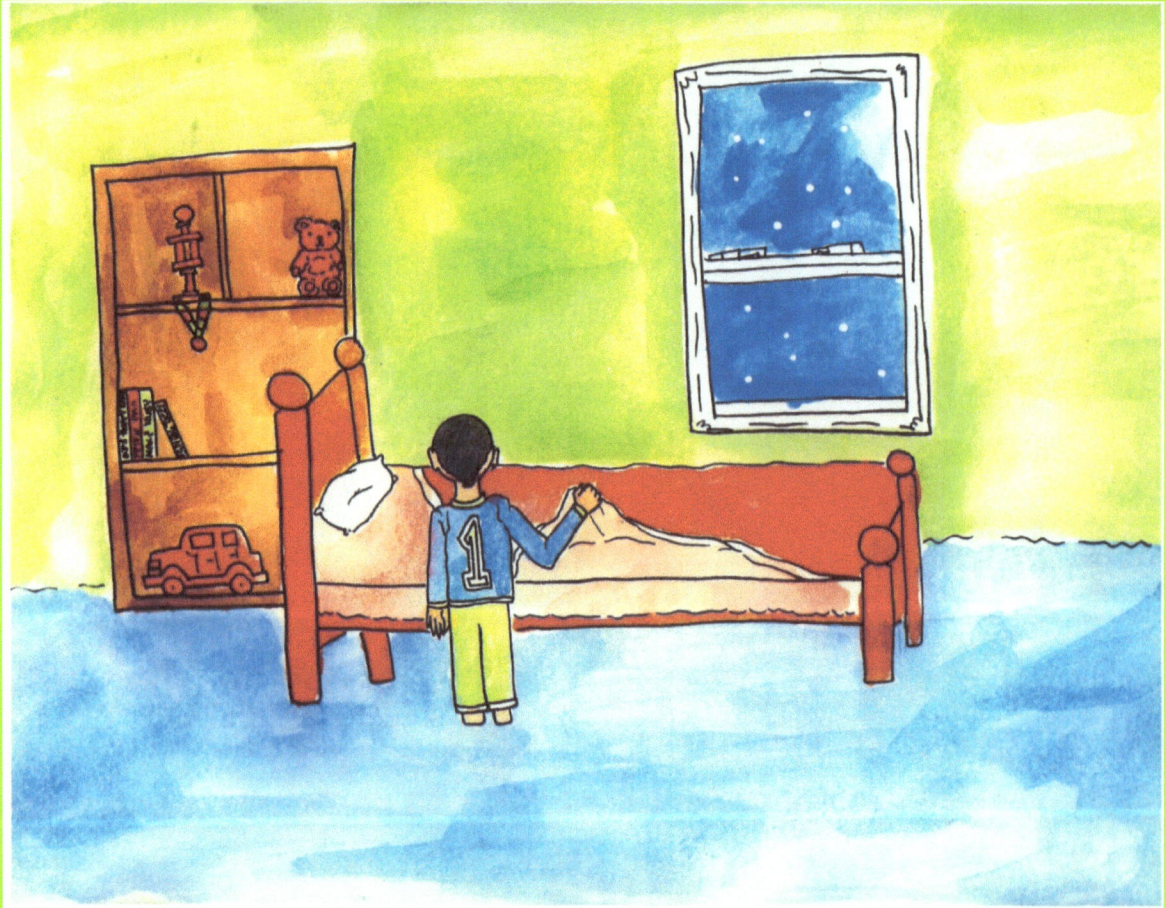

He jumped on the stool and looked in the mirror and smiled. Looking in the mirror, he opened his mouth really big and said, "I love you guys so much." D. J.'s best buddies are his teeth.

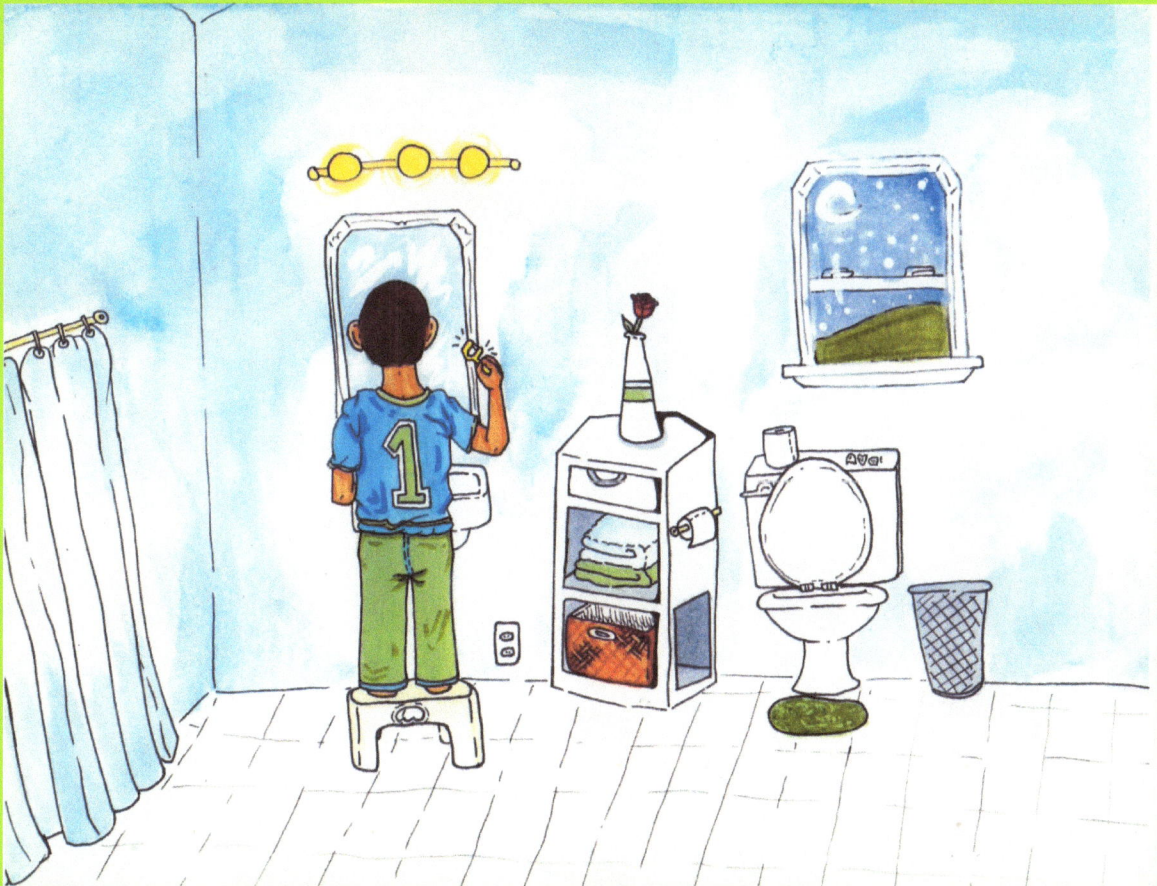

D. J. loves his teeth so much that he has named them. Let me introduce them to you.

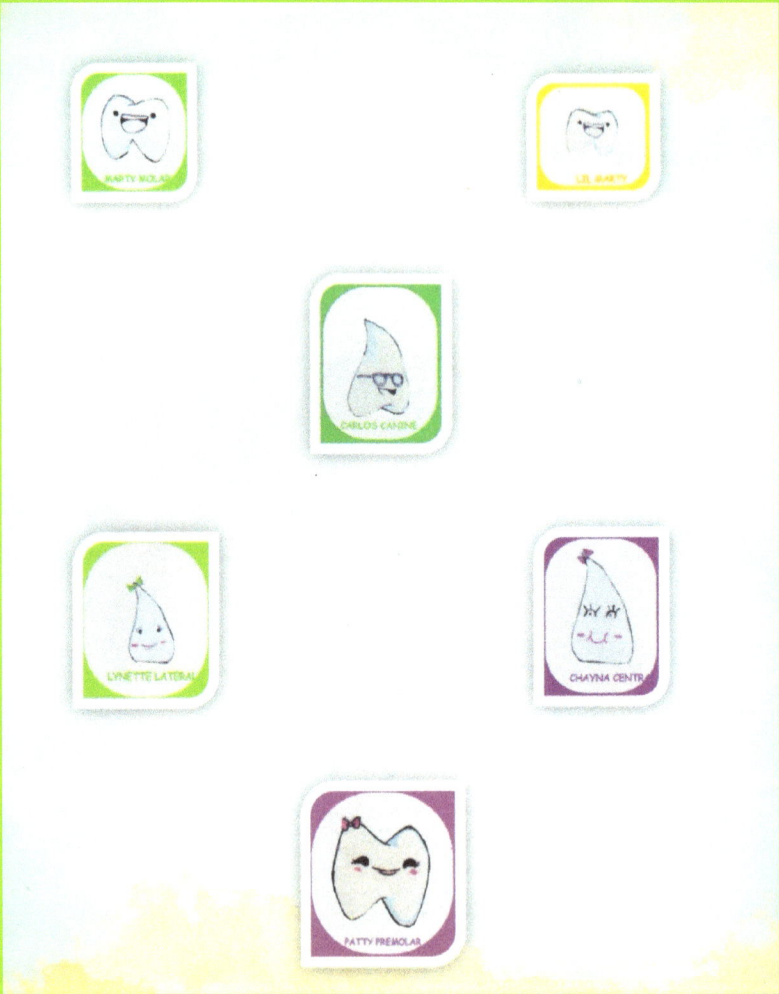

There are four Patty Premolars, four Lynette Laterals and four Chayna Centrals.

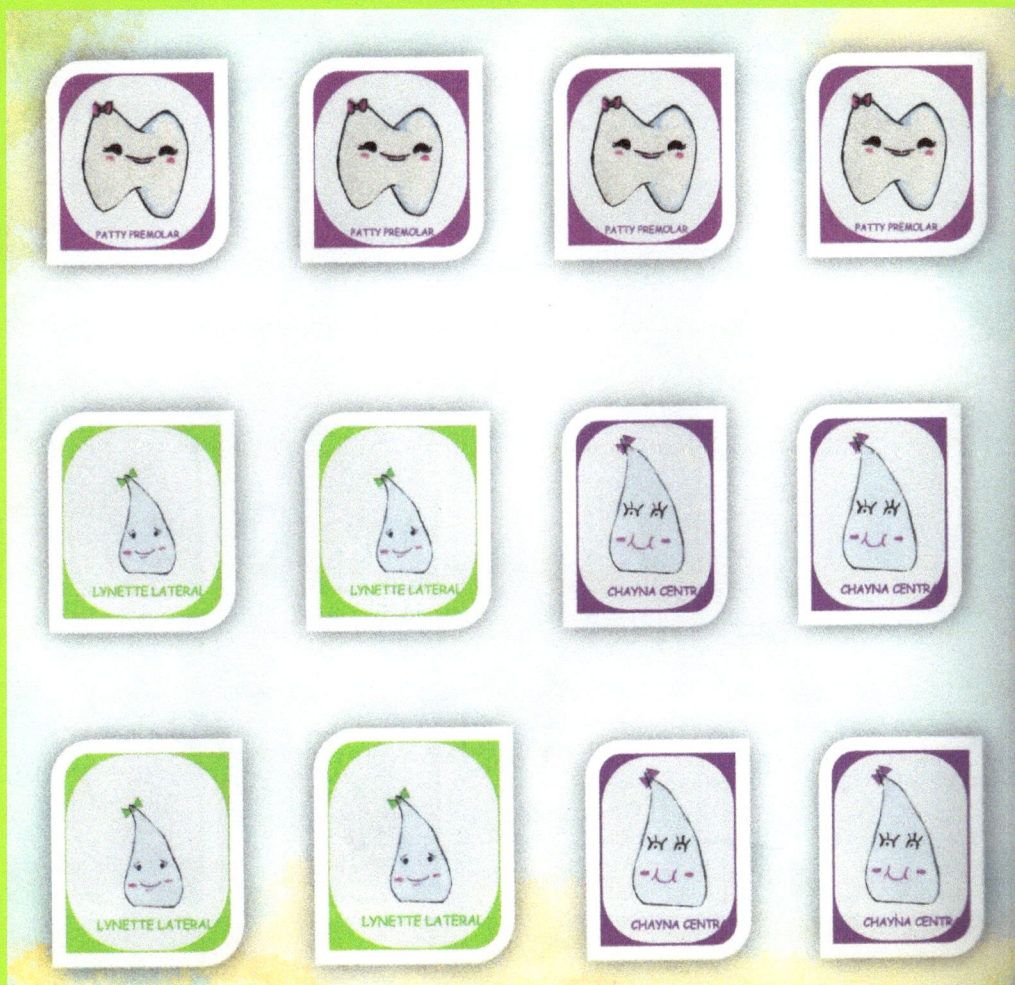

There are four Marty Molars, four Lil Marty's and four Carlos Canine.

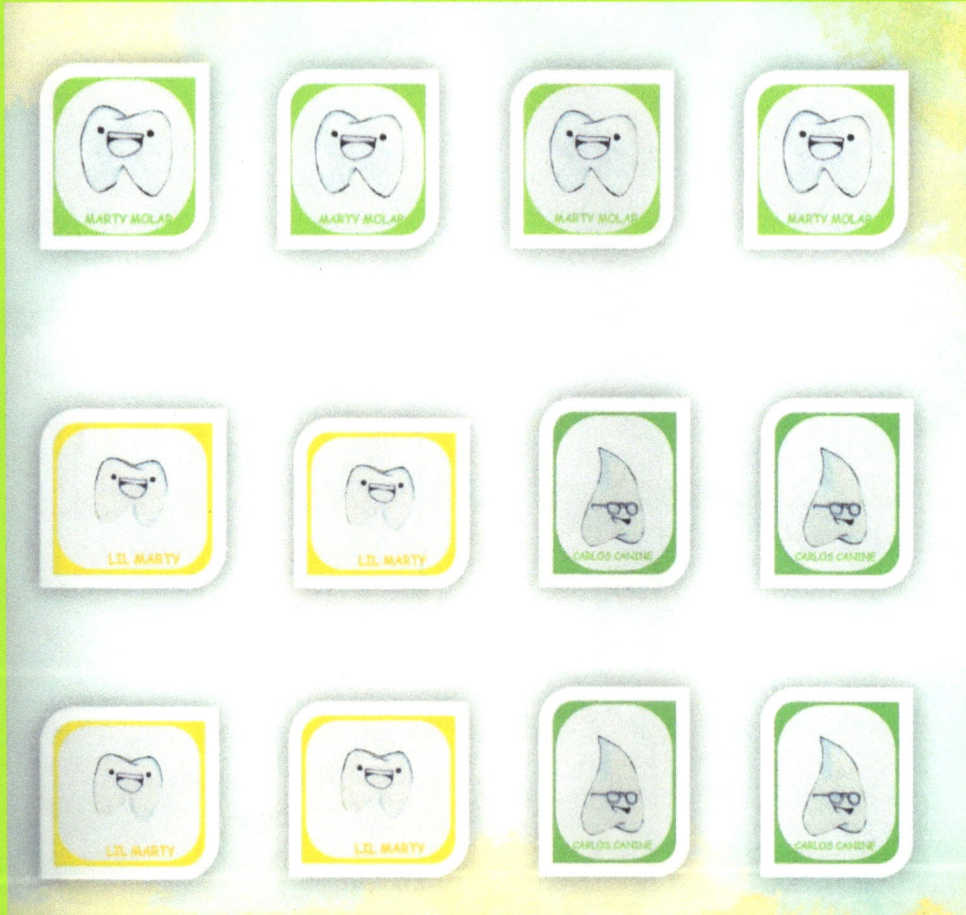

As he picked up his floss pick, he looked at Marty Molar and Lil Marty and said, "I love you guys so much that I'm going to floss every night to get rid of those plaque bugs."

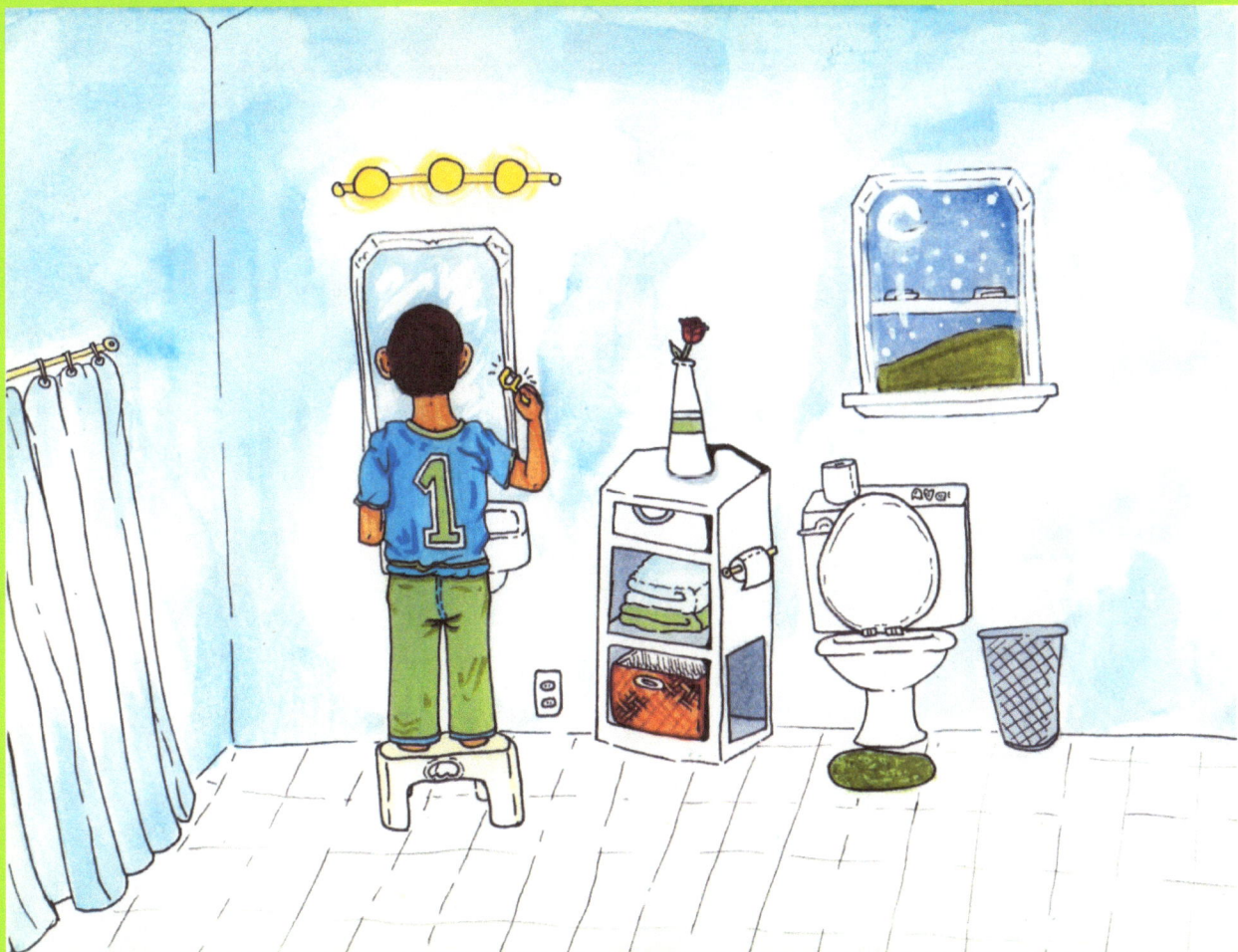

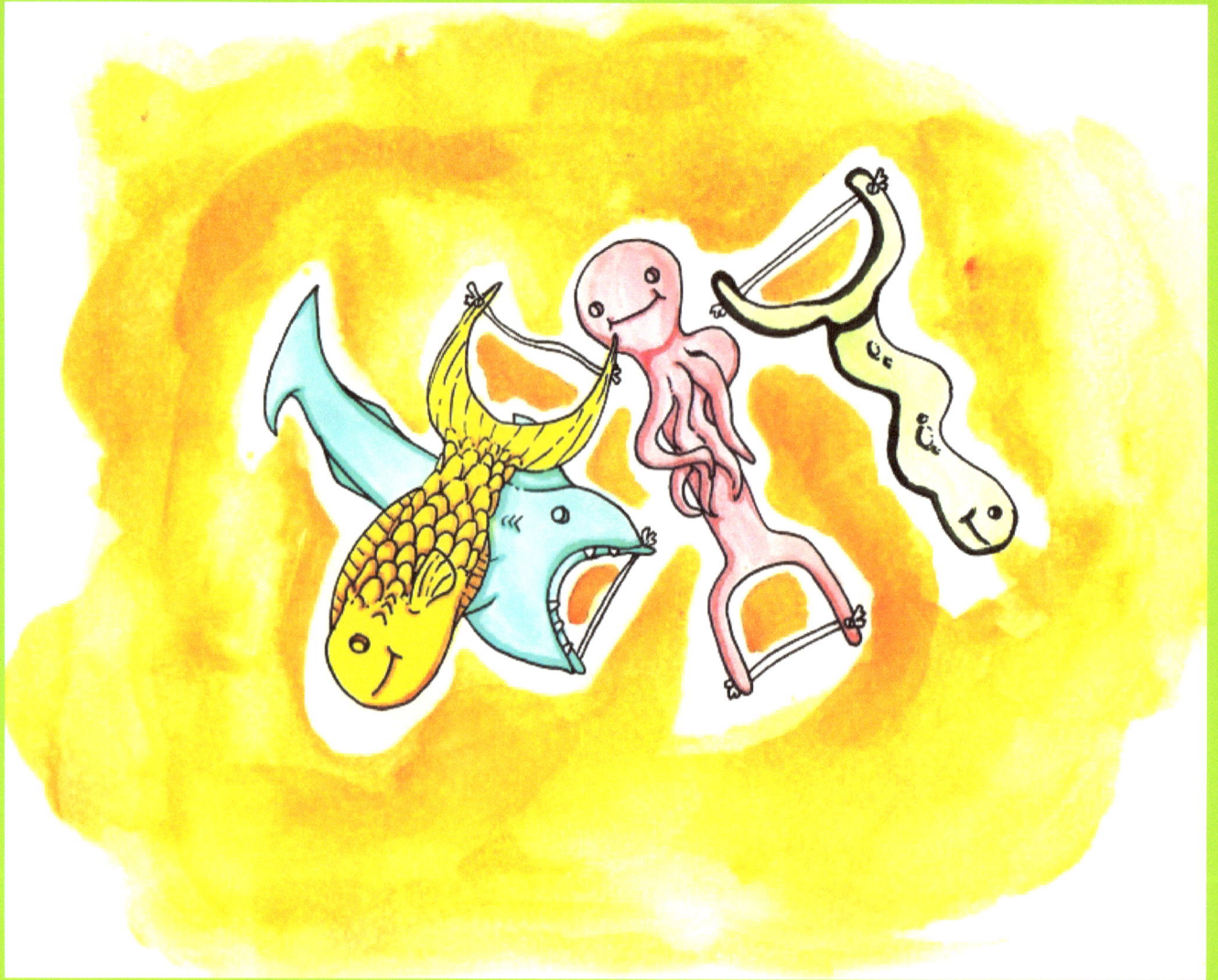

And they said, "We love you so much that we are going to chew your food up very well so you will not get indigestion and hurt your tummy."

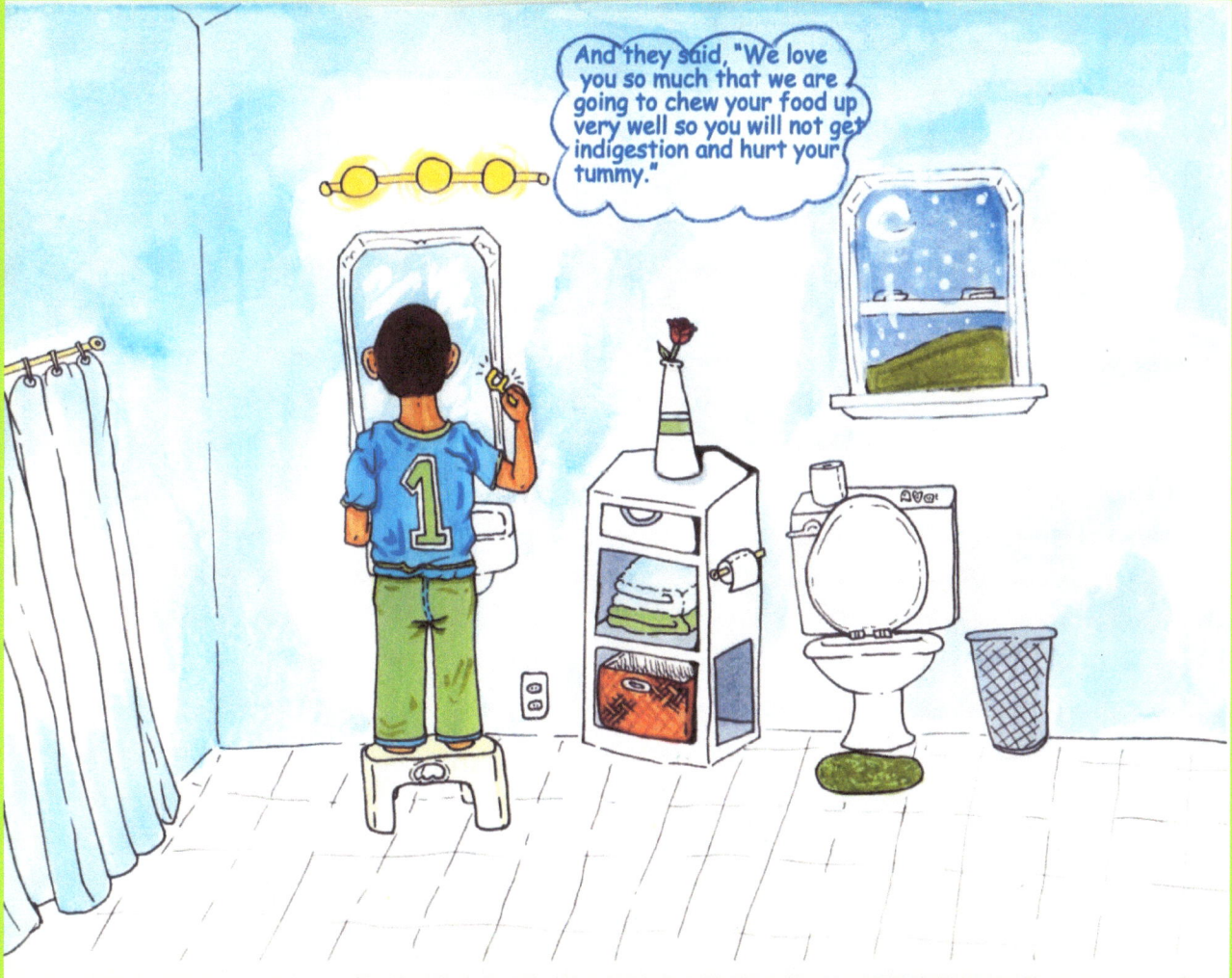

D. J. looked at Marty and Lil Marty and smiled really big. He is so glad that he has a special coating covering them, called sealants. They protect his teeth from bad plaque bugs.

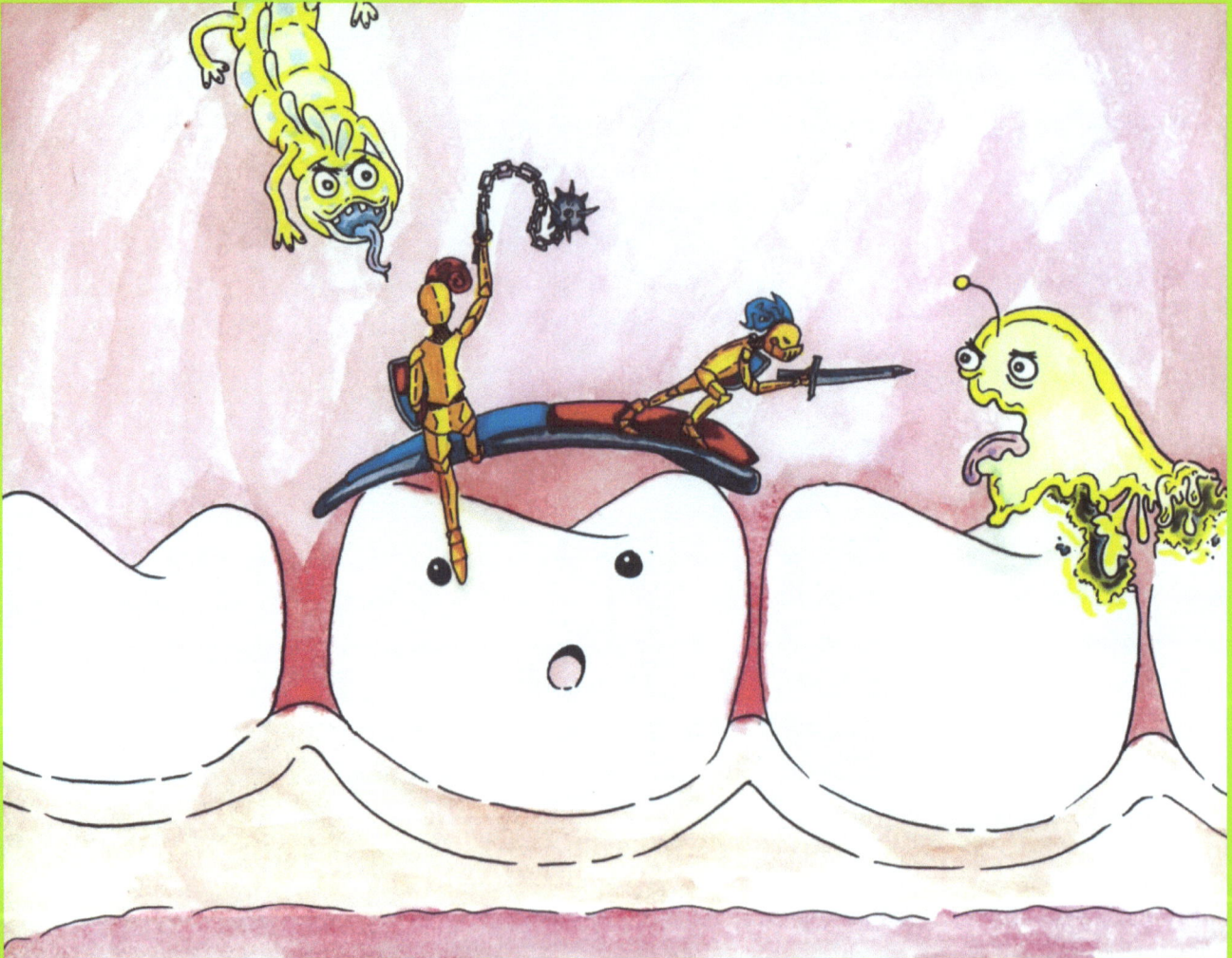

D. J. picked up the rinse and said to Carlos Canine, "I love you so much that I'm going to rinse the bug s off twice a day before and after I brush with a mouth rinse that has these three special letters on the bottle: ADA."

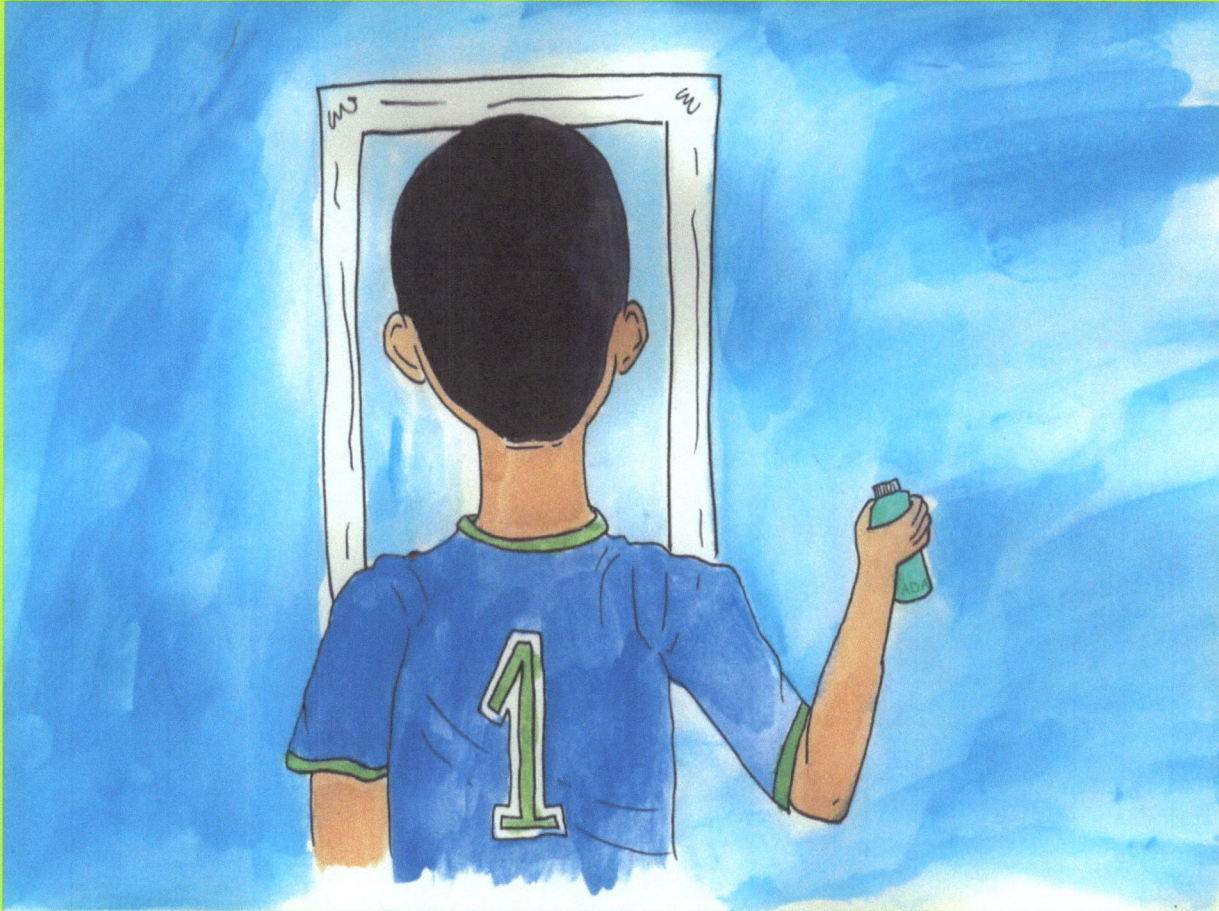

Carlos Canine said to D. J. "We love you so much that we are going to tear your food into small pieces so that the molars can squeeze and chew them up before you swallow it."

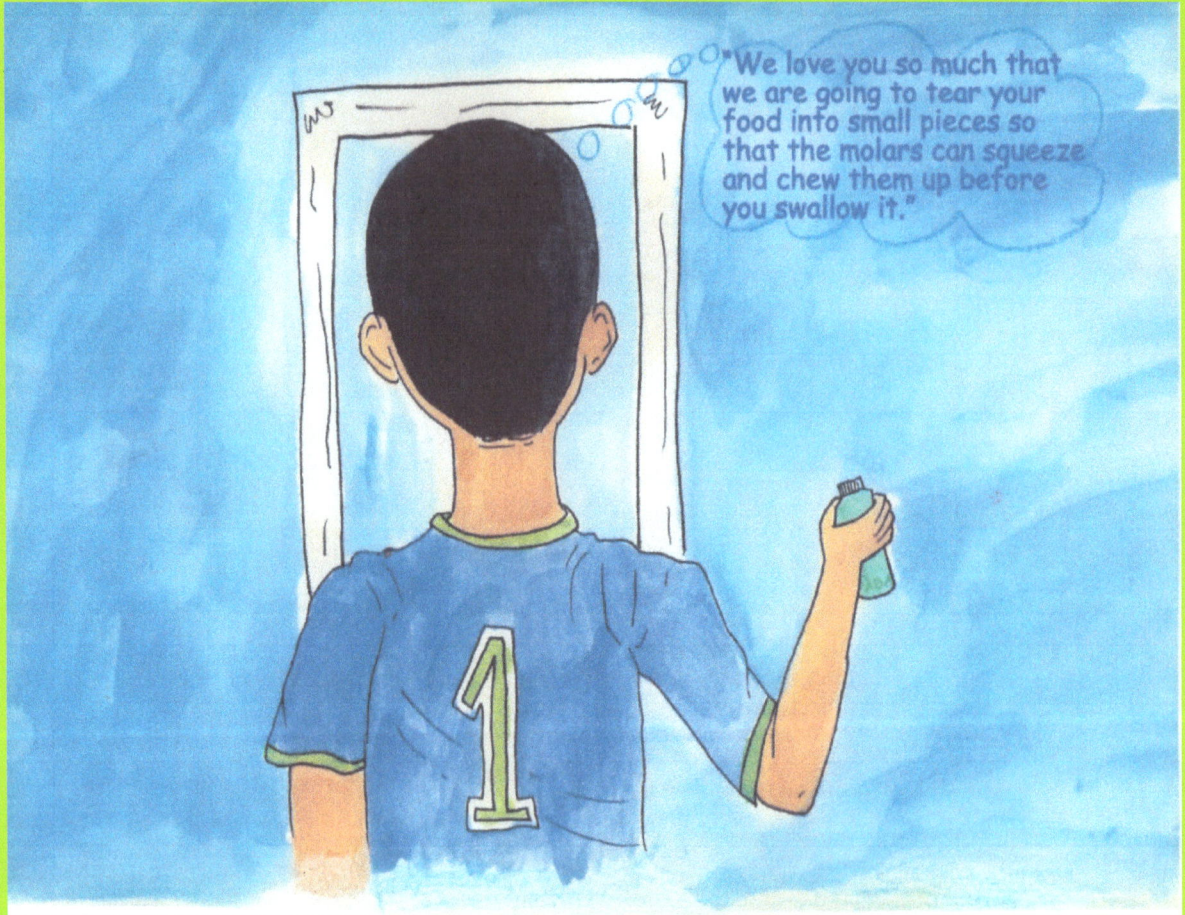

D. J. picked up his toothbrush and toothpaste, looked in the mirror, and smiled really big. His toothbrush and toothpaste had those special letters on them: ADA.

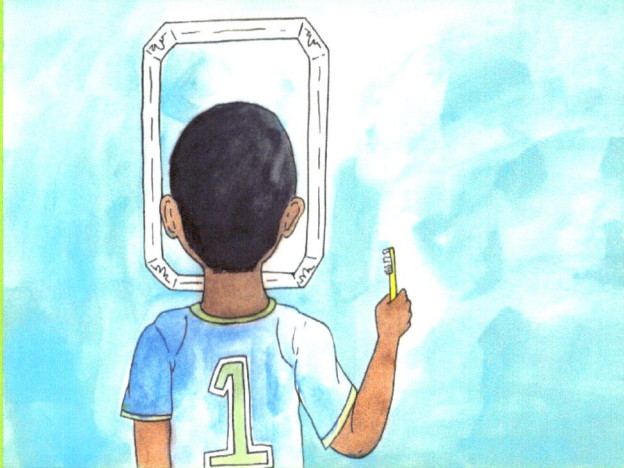

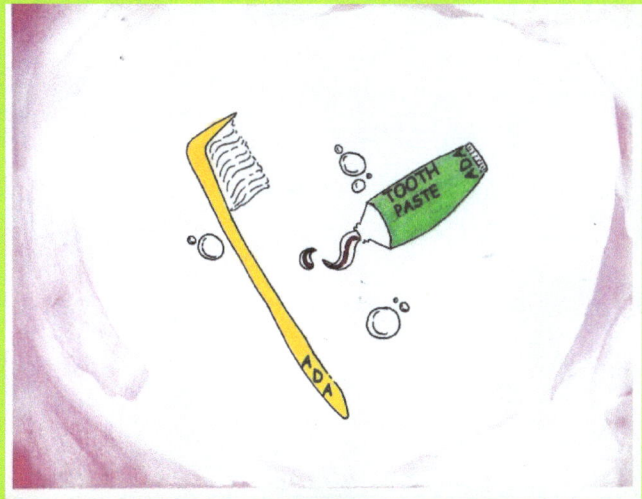

He loves his front teeth so much, and he always gets a lot of compliments about how perfect and beautiful his front teeth are. They are perfect! D. J.'s teeth are just the right shape, they have just the right space, and they are just the right size.

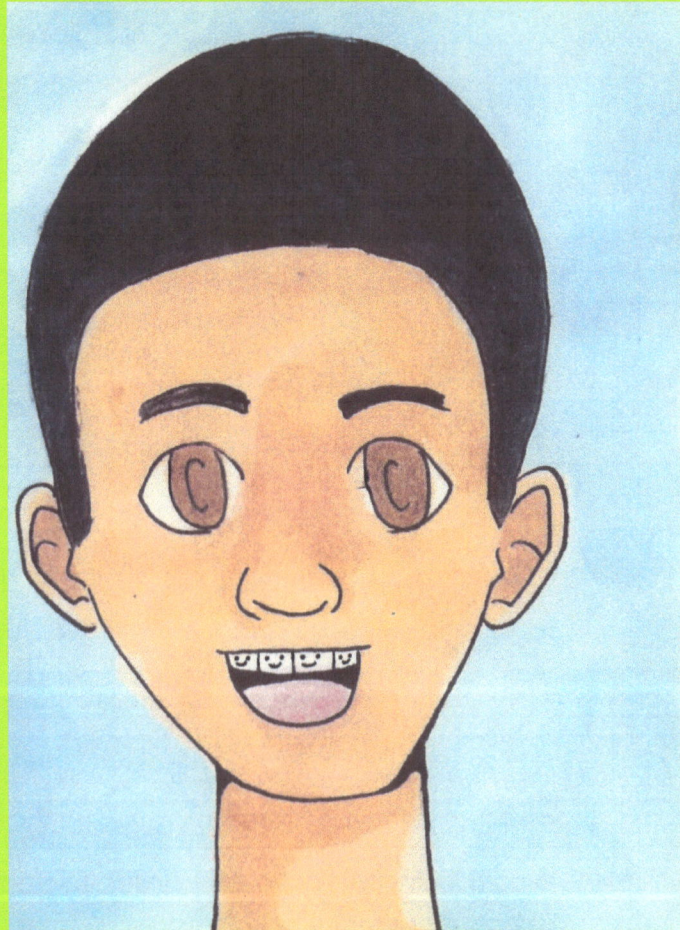

D. J. looked at his teeth and said, "I love you so much. I'm going to eat healthy snacks like fruits and vegetables and limit them during the day."

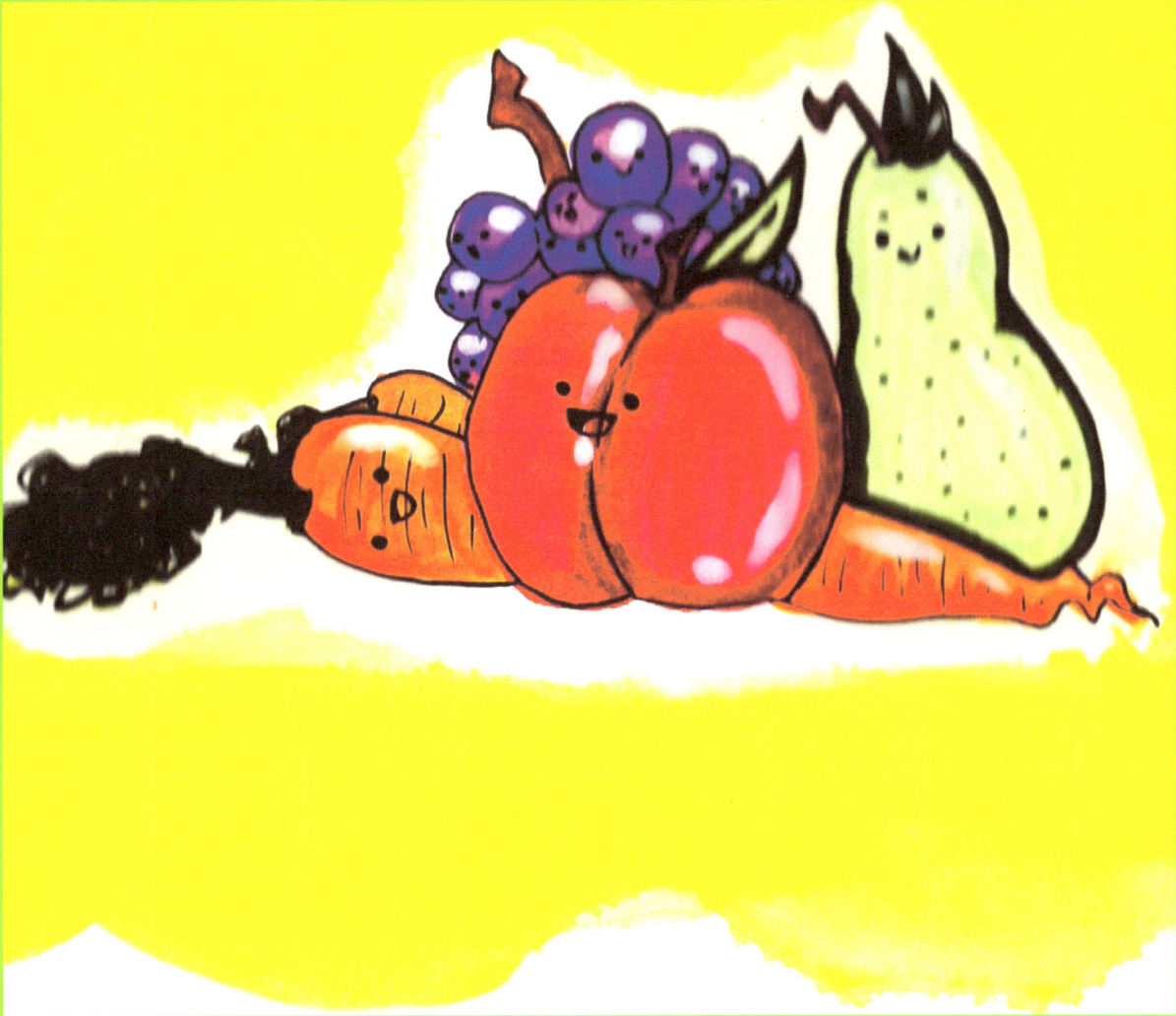

"And I'm not going to eat a lot of candy or drink a lot of sugary drinks. The plaque bugs would eat holes in my teeth if I did."

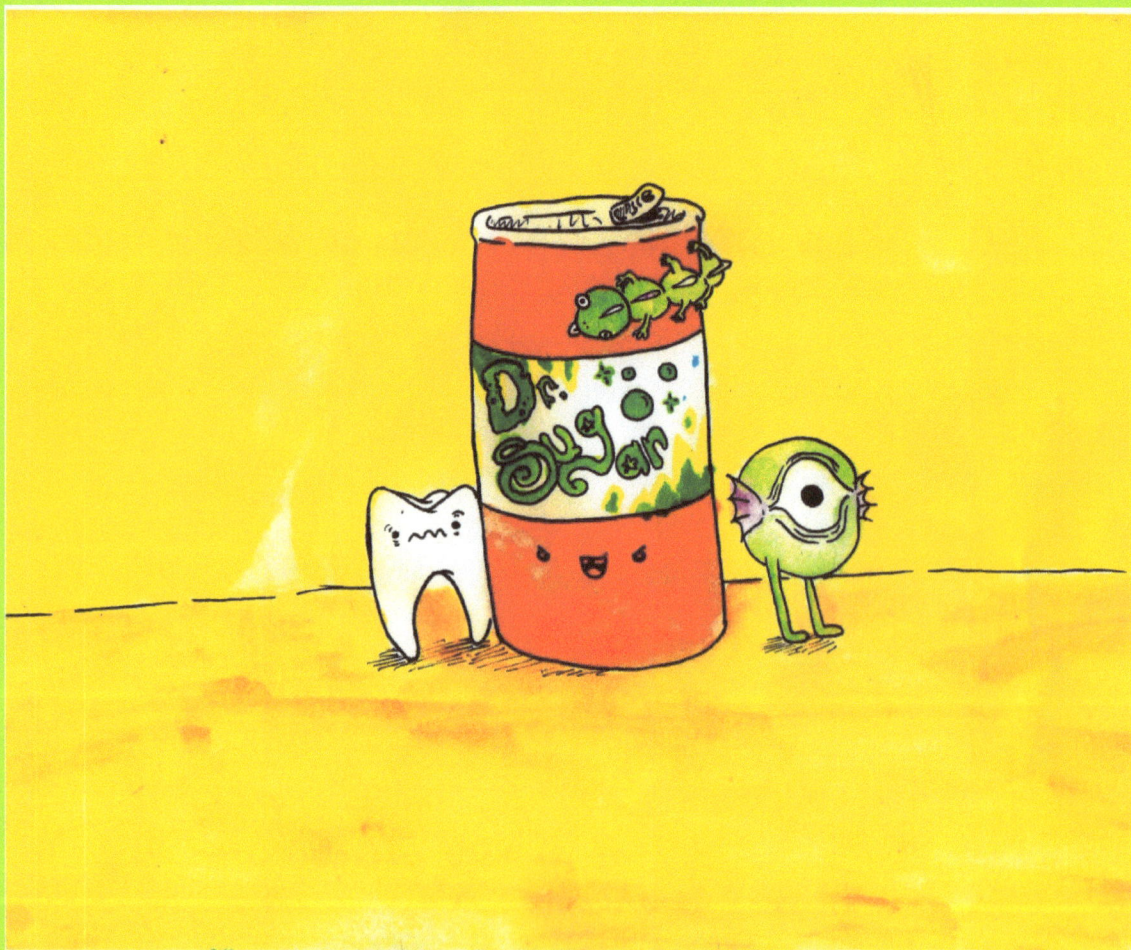

He always starts brushing in the front. Then he brushes the left side, comes back to the right side, and then he brushes the inside of the right teeth and then the left side.

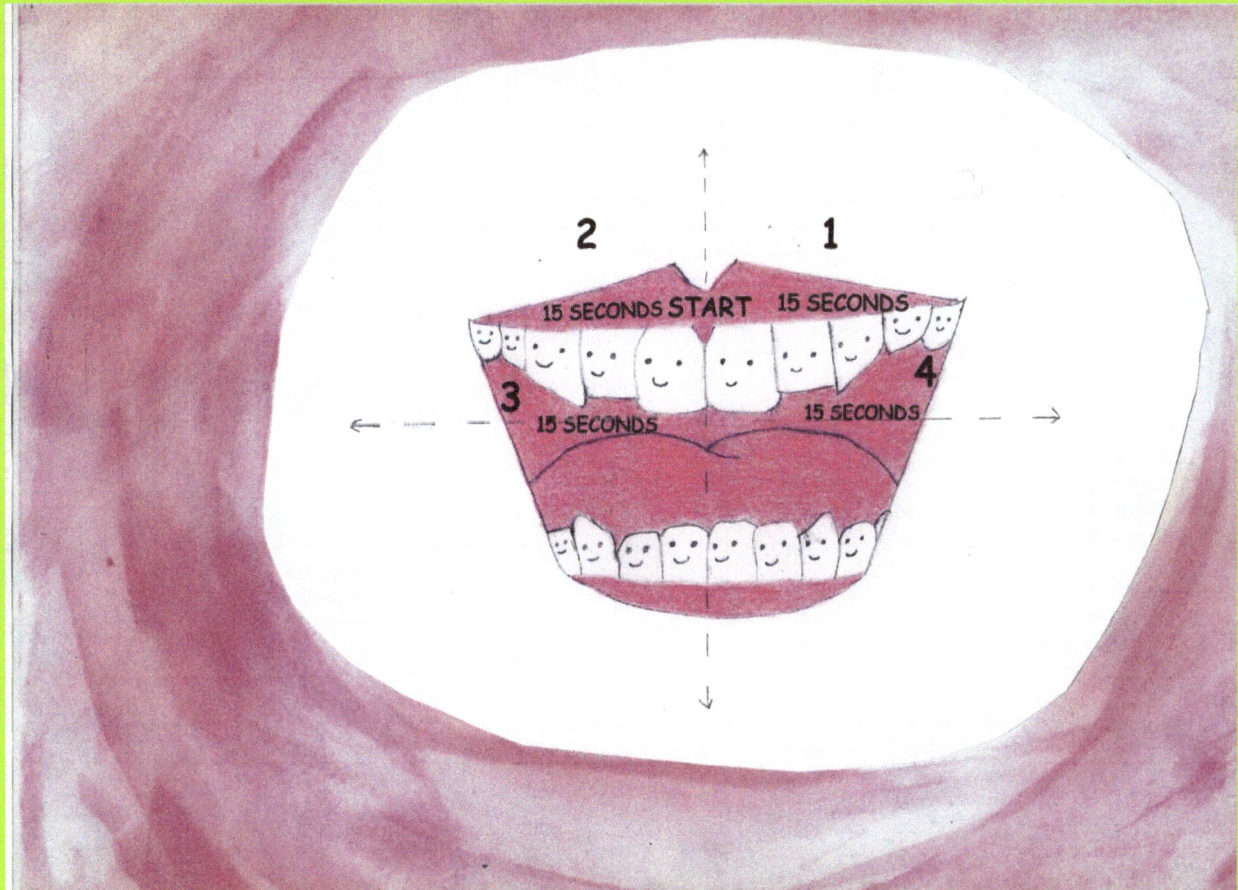

And he continues brushing the lower teeth in the same manner until he is finished. He counts to fifteen in each quadrant, inside and outside.

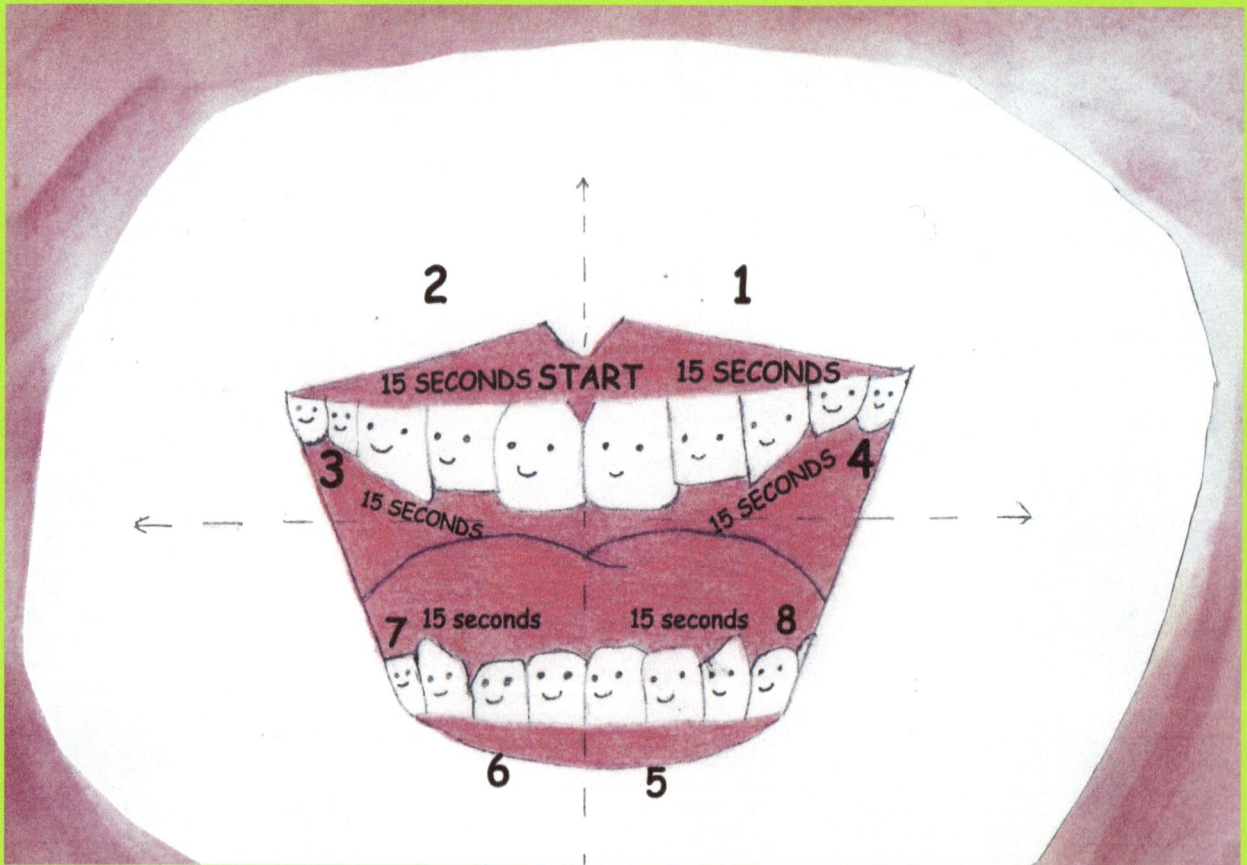

So, he spends two minutes brushing morning and nights. If he's taking pictures or going on a field trip, he spends an extra fifteen seconds on his front teeth at night. He likes for them to sparkle!

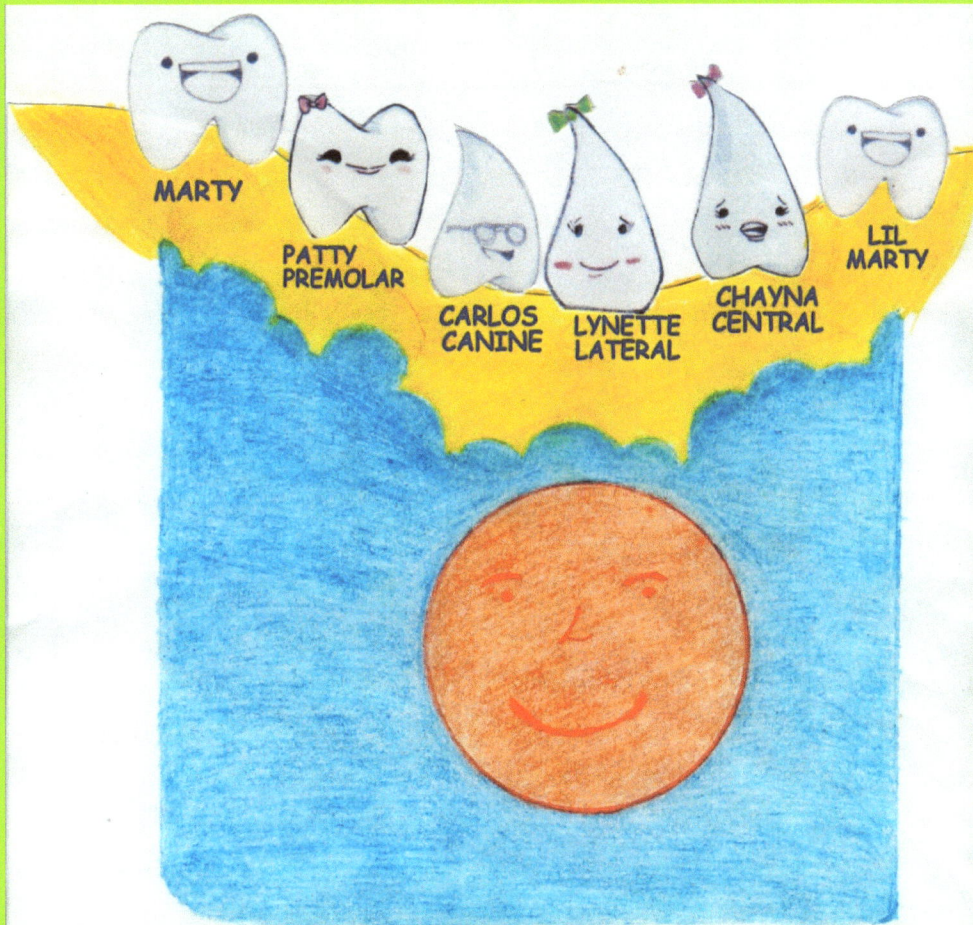

MARTY
PATTY PREMOLAR
CARLOS CANINE
LYNETTE LATERAL
CHAYNA CENTRAL
LIL MARTY

When D. J. finished brushing his teeth, he looked at his teeth and said, "I will make sure I go to my dental team two times a year.

Dental Team:

Dentist and Dental Assistant

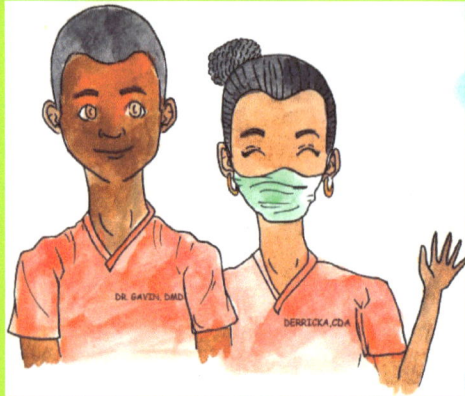

Dental Hygienist

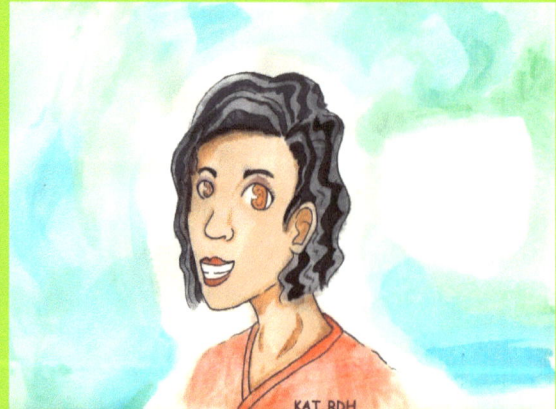

20

D. J. said, "They will make sure I'm doing a good job brushing and keeping you guys clean. You guys are very blessed that my mommy is my dental hygienist.

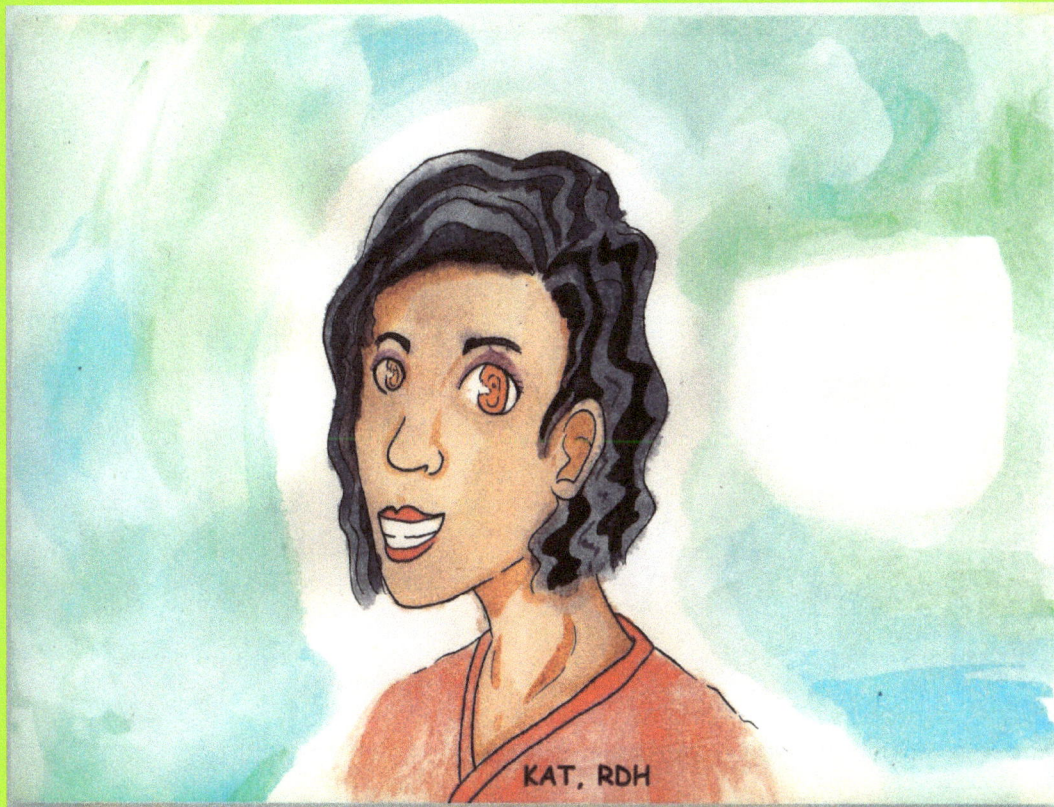

KAT, RDH

As D. J. rinsed his teeth for the second time after he brushed, he yawned. He could hardly keep his eyes open. He had once again spent too much time with his buddies.

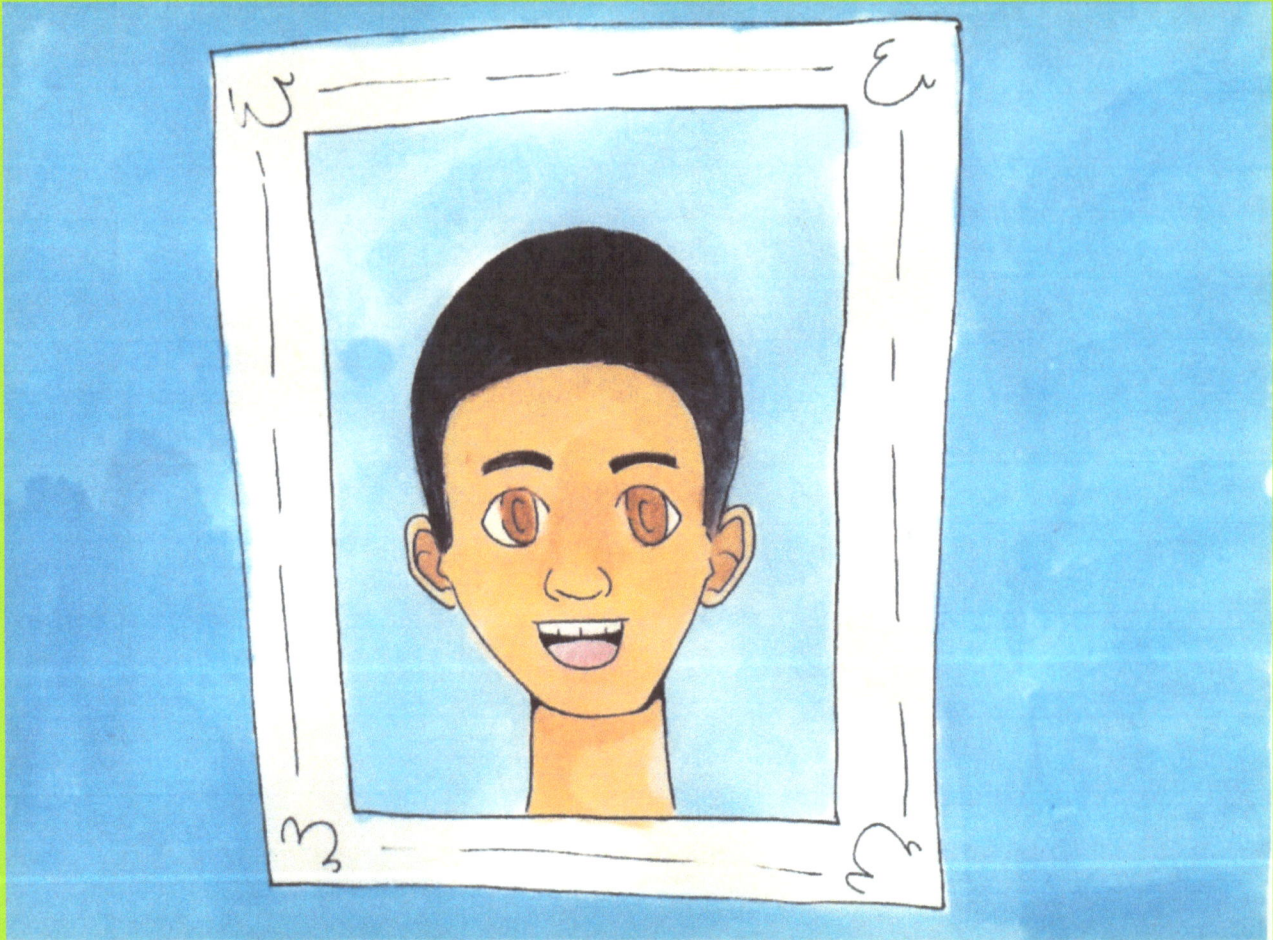

He checked them all one by one, as he did every night, and then crawled into bed.

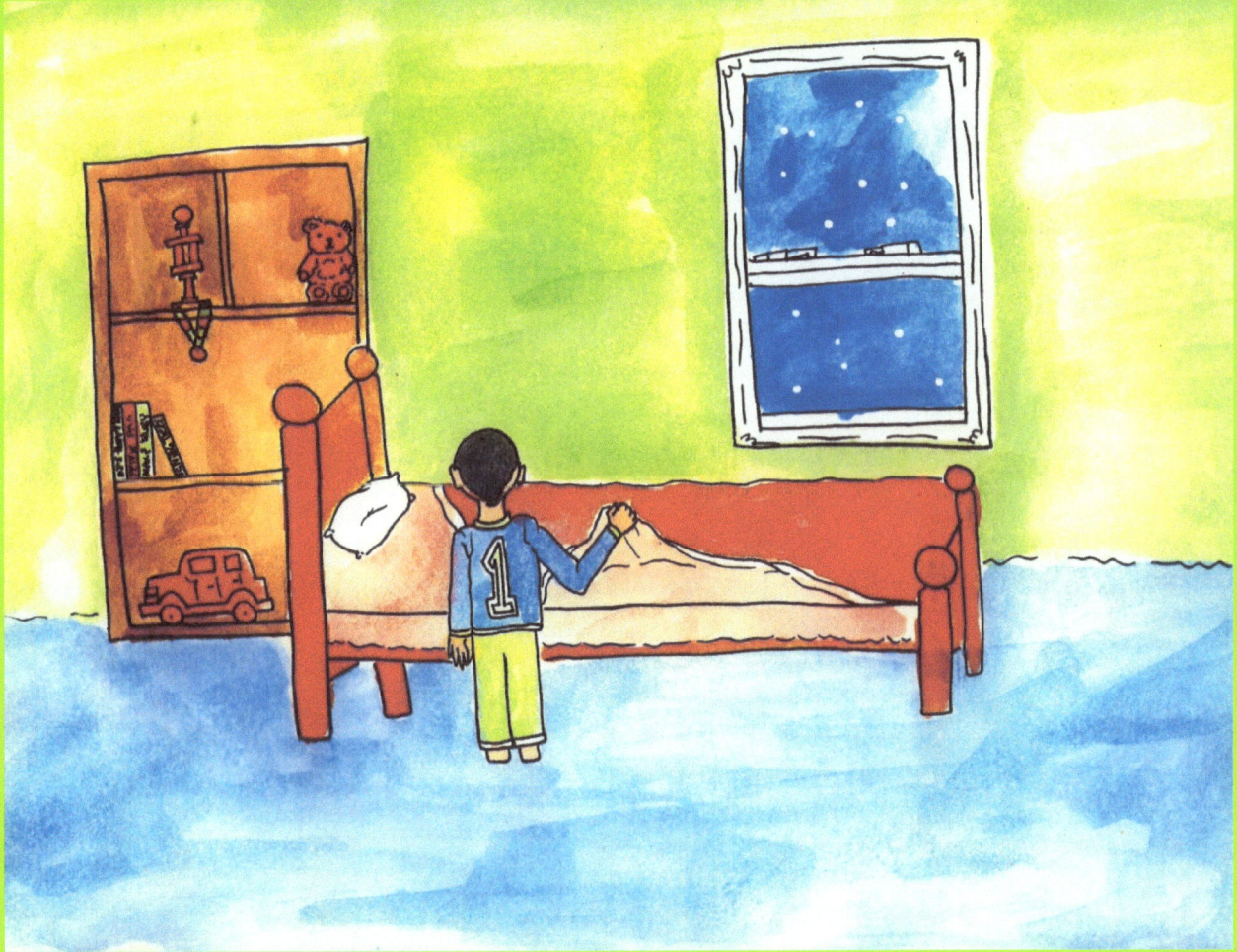

But tonight he got a surprise. One of his front teeth was loose.

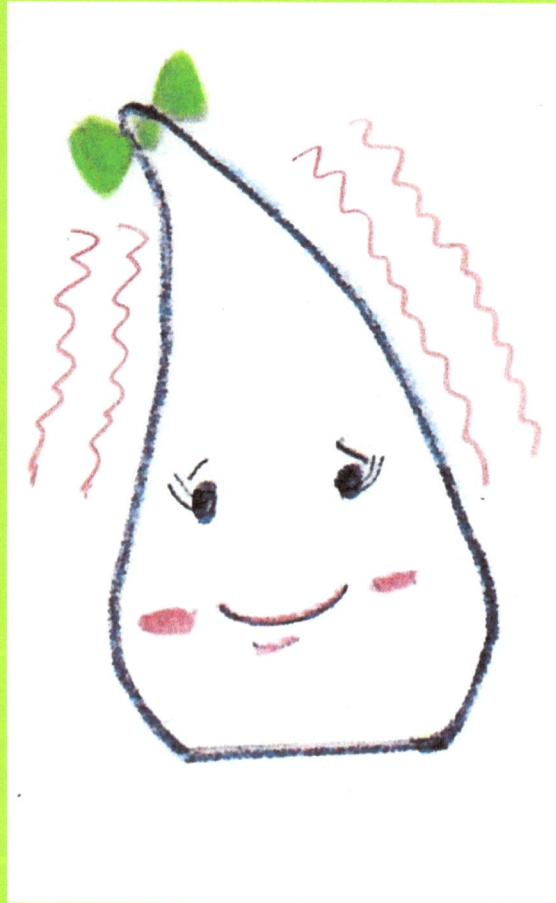

LYNETTE LATERAL

24

He smiled really big and said, "I'm going to take care of you guys for the rest of my life." All of his teeth said, "We are going to chew, tear, and smile for you until the tooth fairy comes to take us to tooth heaven."

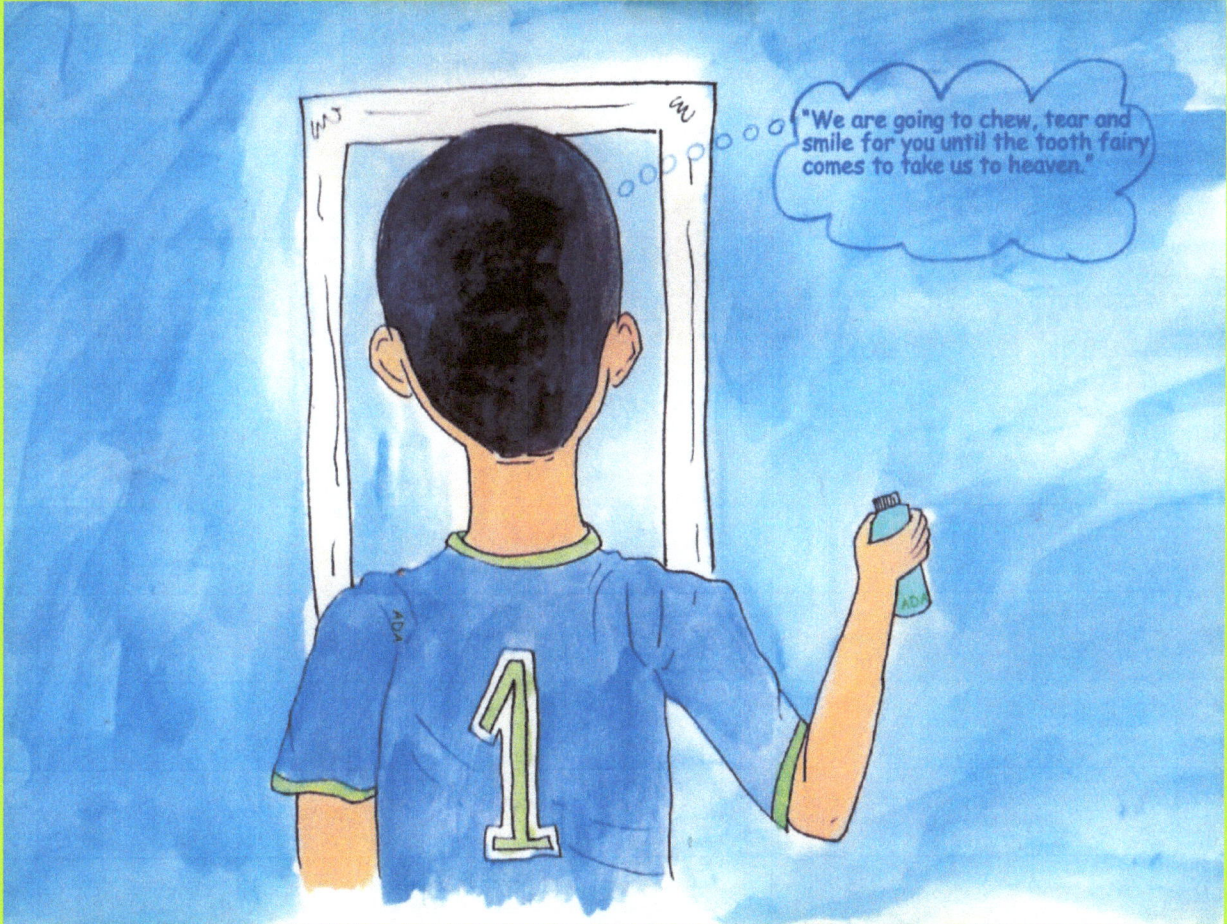

That night, D. J. dreamt of the tooth fairy coming to visit him.

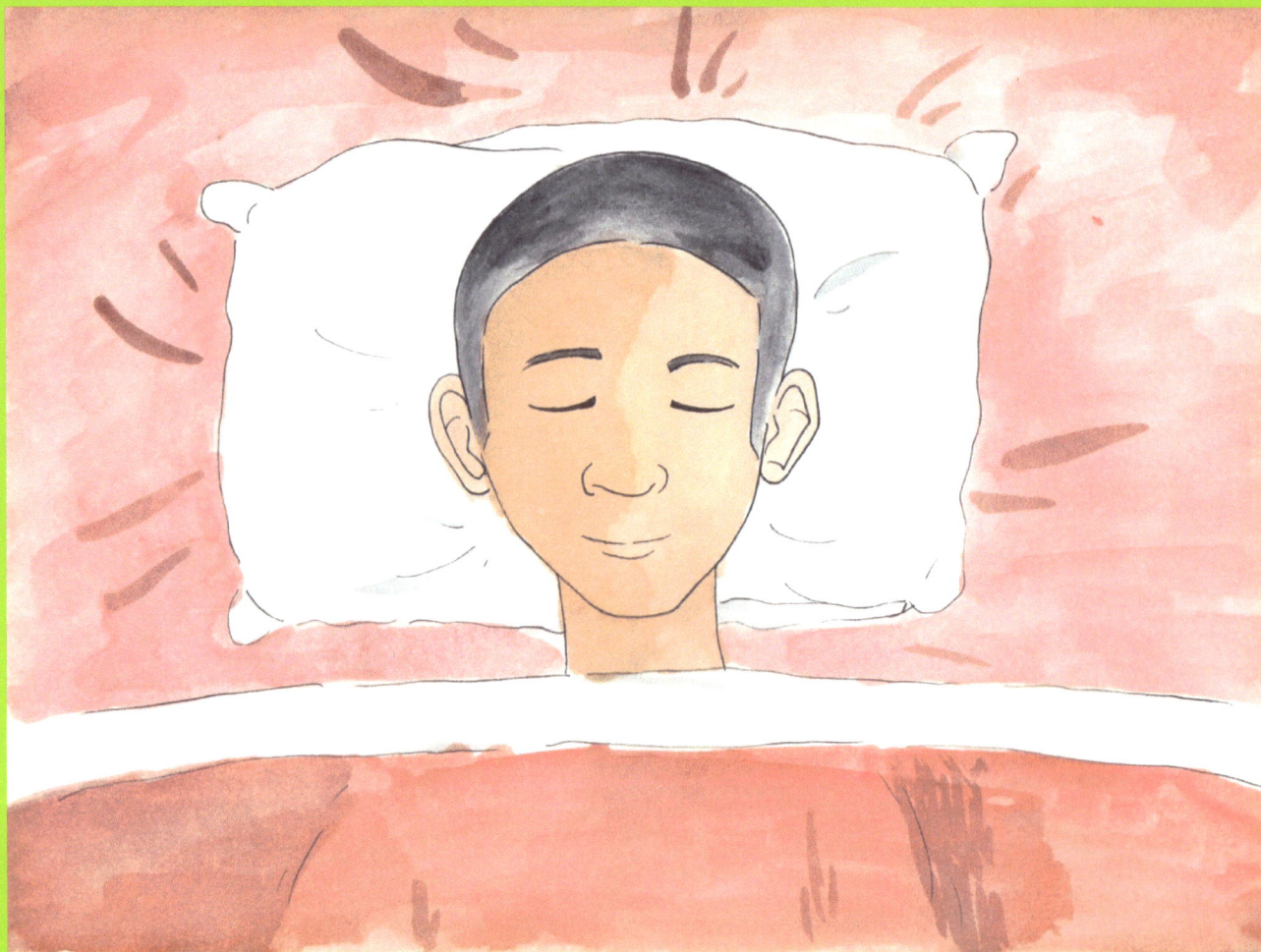

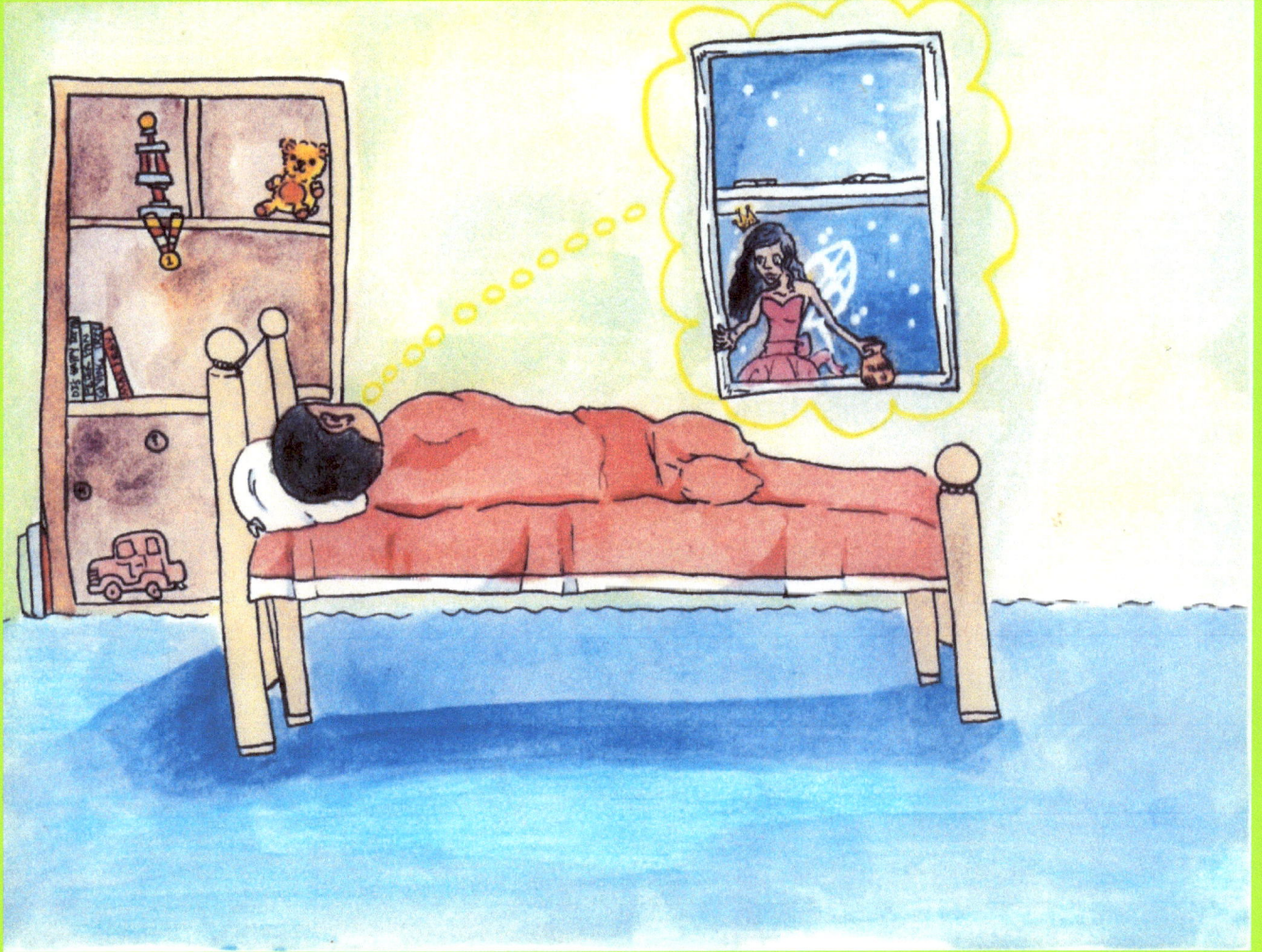

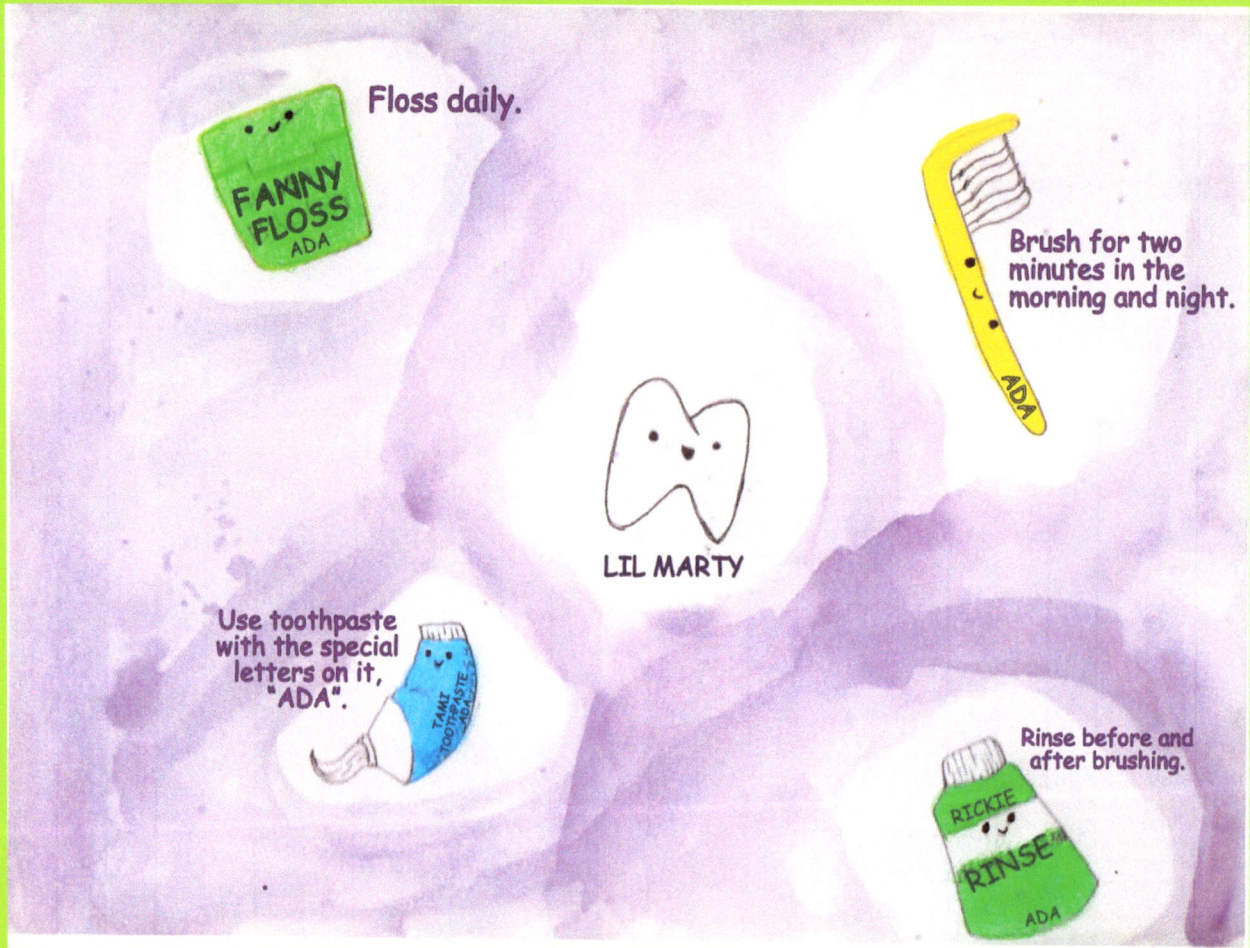

Floss daily.

FANNY FLOSS
ADA

Brush for two minutes in the morning and night.

ADA

LIL MARTY

Use toothpaste with the special letters on it, "ADA".

TAME TOOTHPASTE ADA

Rinse before and after brushing.

RICKIE "RINSE"
ADA

Remember to visit your dental team two times a year and your toothbrush, floss, toothpaste and rinse should always have three special letters on them, ADA.

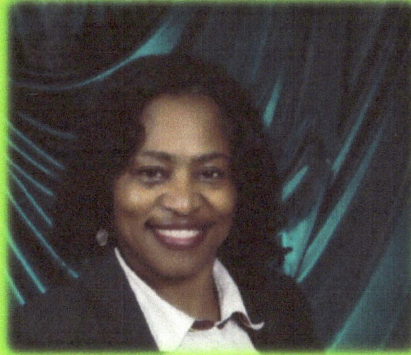

About the Author

She is a native of Summerville, South Carolina. She graduated from Medical University of South Carolina in 1986 with a Bachelor's of Science Degree in Dental Hygiene and graduated from CTU Online in 2009 with an MBA in Health Care Management. She has been married to her elementary school sweetheart for nearly 30 years. They have five children and five grandchildren. Katrina has been a dental hygienist and a health care educator for nearly 30 years. Although her passion has been in the dental field, she has always wanted to write a book. She decided to write a children's dental health book. Her son D. J. had a very vivid imagination as a child and inspired her to write "D. J.'s Happy Teeth." Watch for "D. J.'s Rules for Playing Sports" and "D. J. Gets Braces".

DRAW A PICTURE OF D. J. AND HIS BUDDIES

www.ingramcontent.com/pod-product-compliance
Lightning Source LLC
Chambersburg PA
CBHW060836270326
41933CB00002B/105